S0-ATL-931

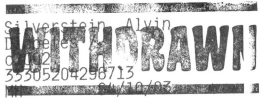
Silverstein, Alvin
WITHDRAWN
3330520429 6713
04/10/03

Diabetes

Dr. Alvin Silverstein,

Virginia Silverstein, and

Laura Silverstein Nunn

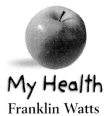

My Health

Franklin Watts

A Division of Scholastic Inc.

New York • Toronto • London • Auckland • Sydney

Mexico City • New Delhi • Hong Kong

SANTA CLARA COUNTY LIBRARY
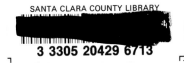

3 3305 20429 6713

Photographs © 2002: Corbis Images/Japack Company: 35; Photo Researchers, NY: 10 (John Bavosi/SPL), 29 (Rainer Berg/OKAPIA), 11 (BSIP/Carlo/Vero/SS), 12 (Ken Cavanagh), 19 (CC Studio/SPL), 18, 27, 31 (Mark Clarke/SPL), 32 (Russell D. Curtis), 8 (Brian Evans), 4 (EXROY-Explorer), 9 (Cecil Fox/SS), 37 (Michael P. Gadomski), 20 (Grantpix), 23 (David M. Grossman), 7 (Joyce Photography), 14 (J.L. Klein & M.L. Hubert/OKAPIA), 21 (Dr. Kari Lounatmaa/SPL), 40 (Larry Mulvehill), 25 (Blair Seitz), 30 (SIU); PhotoEdit: 13 (Frank Siteman), 6 (D. Young-Wolff); The Image Works/Dennis Nett/Syracuse Newspapers: 36; Visuals Unlimited/Nancy P. Alexander: 16.

Cartoons by Rick Stromoski

Library of Congress Cataloging-in-Publication Data

Silverstein, Alvin.
    Diabetes / by Dr. Alvin Silverstein, Virginia Silverstein, and Laura Silverstein Nunn.
        p. (cm).—(My Health)
    Includes bibliographical references and index.
    Summary: Discusses diabetes, its causes and treatments, and emphasizes what can be done to maintain personal health and prevent diabetes attacks.
    ISBN 0-531-12049-X (lib. bdg.)   0-531-16638-4 (pbk.)
    1. Diabetes—Juvenile literature. [1. Diabetes. 2. Diseases.] I. Silverstein, Virginia B. II. Nunn, Laura Silverstein. III. Title. IV. Series.
RC660.5.S55 2002
616.4'62—dc21   2001004965

© 2002 Dr. Alvin Silverstein, Virginia Silverstein, and Laura Silverstein Nunn
All rights reserved. Published simultaneously in Canada.
Printed in the United States of America.
1 2 3 4 5 6 7 8 9 10 R 11 10 09 08 07 06 05 04 03 02

Contents

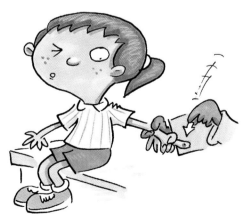

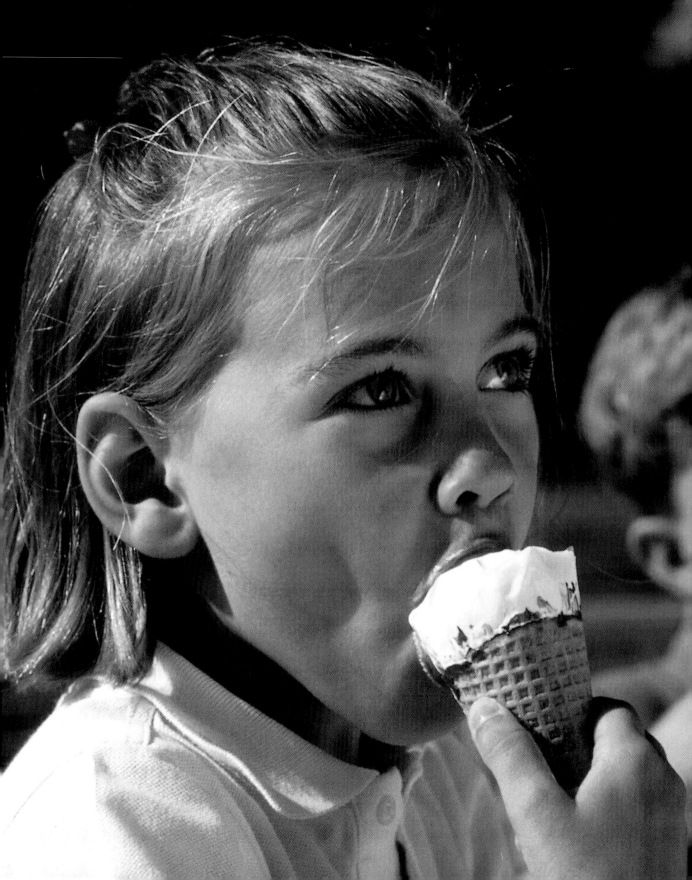

The Sugar Disease

Most kids love to eat sweets. Ice cream, cake, and candy can make a day special, and a sweet dessert after dinner would be a nice treat. Sweet foods usually contain sugar—that's why they taste so good. But eating too many sweets isn't good for anybody. They can rot your teeth and keep you from eating foods that keep you healthy and strong.

For some people, sugary foods are not just unhealthy—they can be dangerous. Normally, your body turns sugar into energy you can use to do everyday activities— play, run, and even think. But some people are not able to use the sugar in their blood properly. They have a condition called **diabetes**. If you have diabetes, sometimes you might feel tired and confused. You might even faint or have to go to the hospital.

◀ **Many kids like to eat ice cream and other sweet foods.**

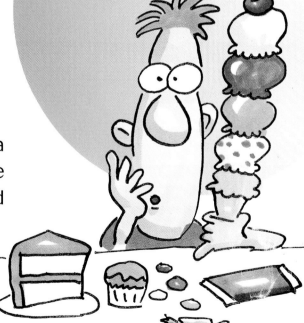

Did You Know...

You can't get diabetes from eating too many sweets.

There is no cure for diabetes, but there are ways to keep the condition under control. Medications can prevent the symptoms. Children usually take a drug that must be injected into the skin. Exercising regularly and eating healthy foods are also important. Blood sugar levels must also be checked regularly. With a good daily routine, a person with diabetes can live a long, healthy life.

Regular exercise will help to keep your body healthy.

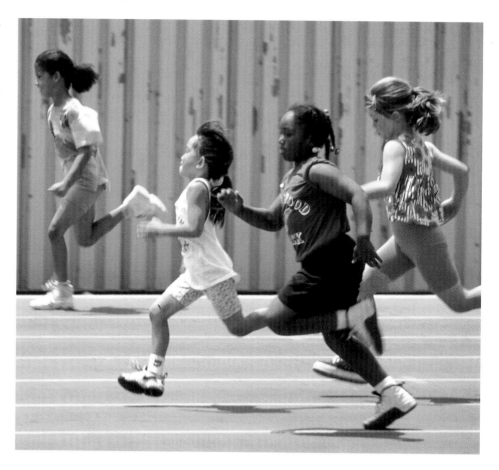

What Is Diabetes?

Diabetes is a disease in which the body cannot use sugar properly, and extra sugar builds up in the blood. Everybody has some sugar in their blood. It supplies the body with energy. But too much sugar in the blood can make you sick.

What Is Sugar?

You probably think of sugar as that white stuff you sprinkle over your cereal or see people put in their coffee or tea. But that is only one kind of sugar. Sugars are found in sweet-tasting foods, such as fruits, candy, and ice cream. They belong to a food group called **carbohydrates**, which are the body's main source of energy. Another type of carbohydrate is **starch**. Starch is made up of a lot of sugar units linked together. Starchy foods include breads, pasta, and rice.

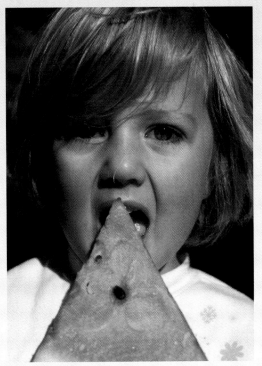

Sugar is found in many foods, including fruit.

Normally, much of the food you eat is turned into a sugar called *glucose*. Some of the glucose is stored, and some of it is used directly for energy. Special chemicals, called *hormones*, are needed for the body to get energy from sugar. These hormones are produced in the *pancreas*, an organ near your stomach.

This diagram shows the organs in the digestive system, including the pancreas.

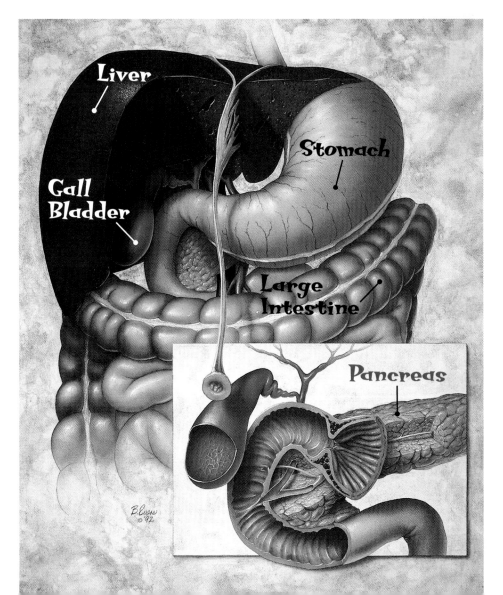

Liver

Stomach

Gall Bladder

Large Intestine

Pancreas

B.Evans ©92

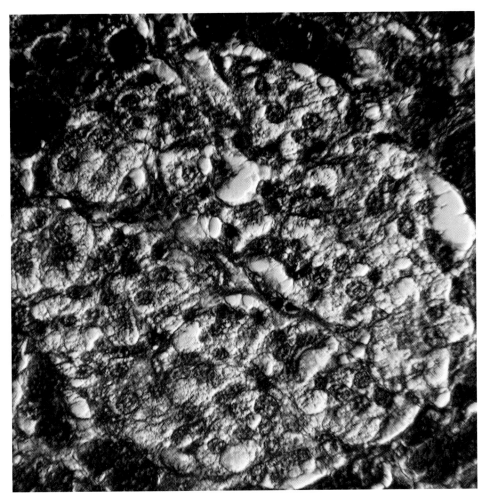

Scattered throughout the pancreas are small blobs of tissue called *islets*. Cells in the islets produce two important hormones, *insulin* and *glucagon*. These hormones are produced all the time. However, the amounts sent out, or *secreted*, from the pancreas depend on how much sugar is in the blood.

Several Functions

The pancreas is a double-duty organ. In addition to secreting insulin and glucose from its islets, it also makes digestive juices. These juices help to break down food so that your body can use it.

This diagram shows how insulin is released from the cell of an islet and passes into the bloodstream.

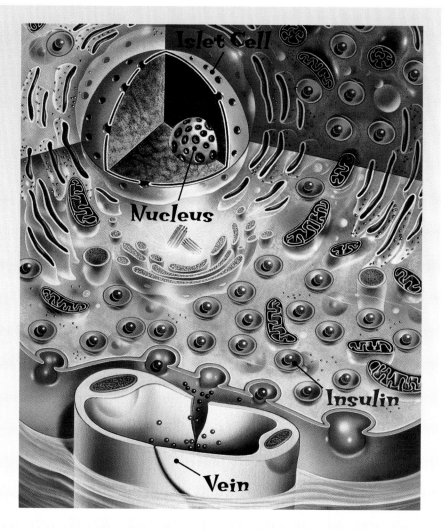

Islet Cell

Nucleus

Insulin

Vein

Both hormones work to control the body's use of sugar, but they have opposite effects on the blood. How do insulin and glucagon work?

After you eat, the foods are **digested**, or broken down in your mouth, stomach, and intestines.

The digestive process changes starches into sugars. Sugars and other food materials pass into your blood. Now it is time for insulin to go into action.

When the amount of sugar in the blood rises, the pancreas secretes insulin. Insulin makes the blood sugar level go down by helping glucose pass out of the blood and into the cells of the body. Some of the sugar in the body cells is used right away to produce energy. Some is changed into starch and fats and stored in the body. Starches and fats are handy forms to store sugar until the body needs some extra energy.

When the blood sugar level falls, the pancreas secretes more glucagon. This hormone makes the blood sugar level go up by causing starch in the

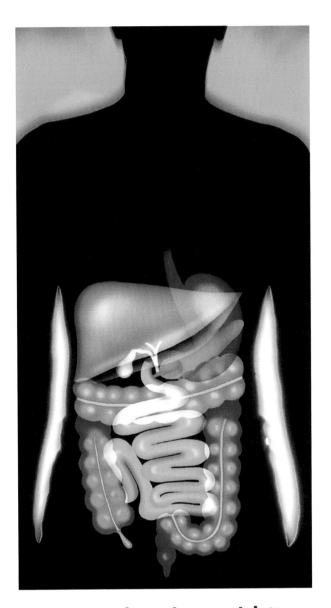

Food passes from the mouth into the stomach, and then on to the intestines to be broken down by digestive juices from the pancreas.

Temporary Diabetes

If you have diabetes, you have to live with it for the rest of your life. You cannot grow out of it. Some pregnant women, however, develop a type of diabetes that disappears after the baby is born. This condition is called **gestational diabetes**, because gestation is another word for pregnancy. Women who develop gestational diabetes have a greater risk for problems during pregnancy, and also for developing diabetes later in their lives.

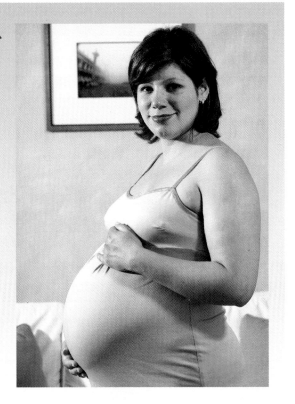

cells to turn back into glucose. The glucose goes into the blood and is then carried to the cells that need energy.

Insulin and glucagon work together like members of a team. They make sure that the amount of sugar in the blood is always just right.

When the body cannot make enough insulin, or cannot use the insulin properly, glucose cannot get into the cells. Eventually, extra sugar builds up in the blood, causing the symptoms of diabetes.

Types of Diabetes

There are two main types of diabetes: type 1 and type 2. Both forms result in too much sugar in the blood and produce similar symptoms. But there are some very important differences between the two forms.

Type 1 diabetes used to be called juvenile diabetes because it affects mainly children, teens, and young adults, but it can occur at any age. In type 1 diabetes, the pancreas no longer produces insulin. This can be very dangerous. Type 1 diabetes can appear suddenly. You may feel fine one day and then very sick the next. It is very important to correct the blood sugar levels quickly to prevent life-threatening complications.

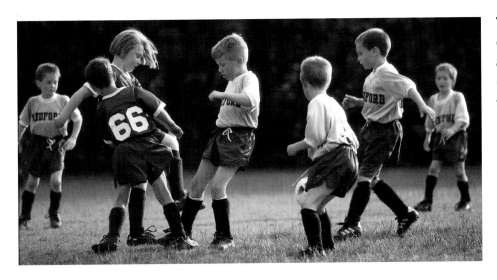

Type 1 diabetes affects mainly children and teenagers.

Type 2 diabetes is the most common form—it accounts for about 90% to 95% of all diabetes cases. It affects mostly adults after the age of forty, although children may also develop this type. In type 2 diabetes, the pancreas does produce insulin. However, it does not produce enough of it, or the body cannot use it properly. As a result, the body cells cannot get energy from sugar. Doctors call this condition **insulin resistance**. This type of diabetes can take years to develop.

In both types of diabetes, the body cells become starved for energy, and symptoms develop. Here are some warning signs of either type of diabetes.

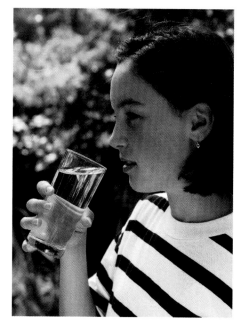

You may:
- be thirsty all the time
- have to **urinate** frequently
- feel weak and tired
- feel hungry all the time
- lose weight, even though you eat a lot
- get sores on your skin that take a long time to heal
- notice that objects look fuzzy or blurry
- have pains in your legs

One sign of diabetes is that you are thirsty all of the time.

Anybody can have some of these warning signs from time to time without having diabetes. But if you have many of these signs, and have them all the time, you should see a doctor.

People who have diabetes have sugar in their urine. How does sugar get in the urine? Urine is made in the kidneys. The kidneys take out waste products from the blood. They also take out some water to flush the wastes away. If there is too much of something in the blood, the kidneys take that out too. People with diabetes have too much sugar in their blood, and soon sugar turns up in their urine.

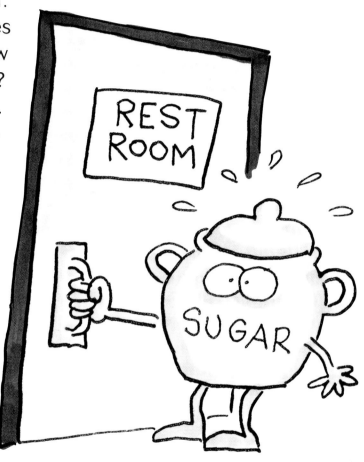

When sugar passes into the urine, the urine gets thicker. Then more water goes from the blood into the urine. This water washes out other things too. Vitamins, minerals, proteins, and fats are lost along with the sugar and water.

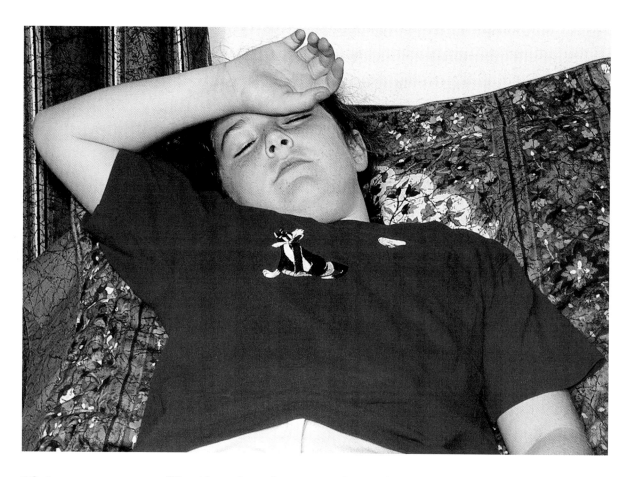

Diabetes may make you feel weak and tired because your body is not able to create the energy it needs.

That's why the warning signs develop. If you have diabetes, your kidneys have to make a lot of urine because they are getting rid of the extra sugar from the blood. So you may have to go to the bathroom a lot. You are also thirsty all the time because you are losing so much water. You feel unusually weak and tired because your body can't use sugar for the energy it needs. You are hungry because you are

What's in a Name?

The name *diabetes* comes from a Greek word meaning "a siphon," a U-shaped tube that transfers liquid from one container to another. Ancient Greek doctors noticed that when people with diabetes drank large amounts of liquid, the fluid seemed to run right through them, as water runs through a siphon, and they would have to urinate often.

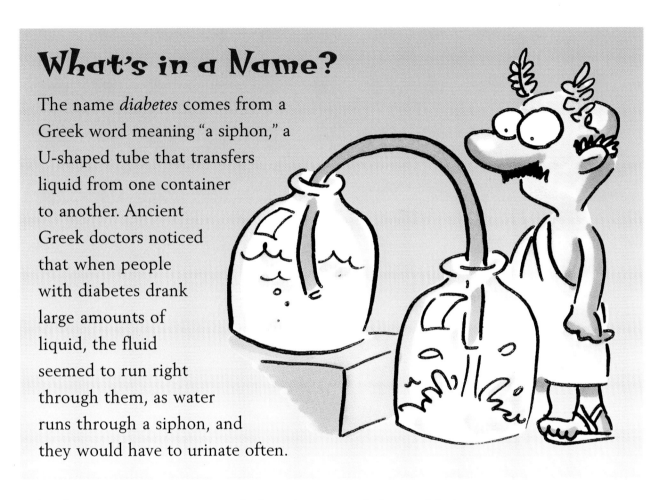

losing so many good food materials, which are getting washed out in your urine.

Too much sugar in the blood can also cause more serious problems. People with diabetes have a high risk of getting heart disease. High blood sugar levels may cause eye problems, possibly even resulting in blindness. Poorly controlled diabetes may also cause dental problems, high blood pressure,

People with diabetes must watch any cuts or scrapes carefully so they do not get infected.

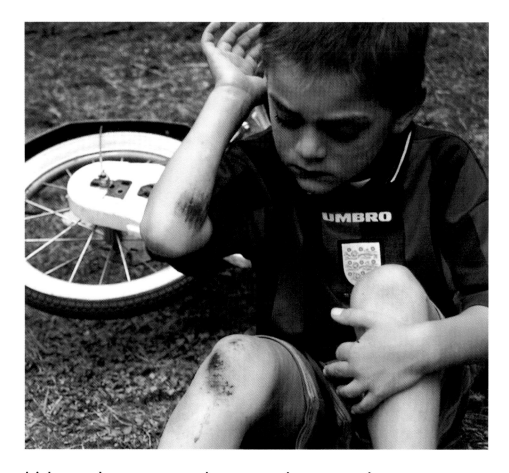

kidney damage, and nerve damage that may produce pain and numbness. Cuts and other wounds of diabetes patients are more likely to get infected than those of people without diabetes, and they do not heal as quickly. Many people with diabetes have problems with their feet, and even small cuts can become serious. In severe cases, sometimes part of the foot may have to be amputated (removed).

What Causes It?

About 16 million Americans have diabetes, and most of them are adults. However, health experts say that more children are getting diabetes than ever before. This may be because many kids today are eating too much food

that is high in fat and sugar, and they are not getting enough exercise. This may result in **obesity**—being extremely overweight. The extra weight is stored as body fat, which can lead to insulin resistance making body cells unable to use insulin effectively. Gaining a lot of weight increases a person's chance for developing type 2 diabetes. There is no link between obesity and type 1 diabetes.

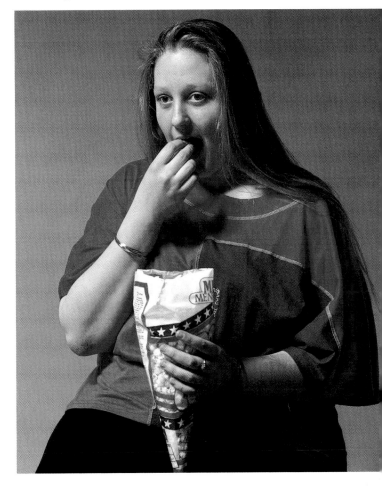

Many kids and teenagers today are eating too much junk food and not getting enough exercise.

Researchers believe that an overweight person is more likely to develop diabetes if someone in his or her family has it. Studies have shown that diabetes can be **inherited** when **genes** are passed down from one generation to another. Certain genes may play an important role in the development of diabetes. But even if someone in your family does have the disease, that doesn't mean you will get it.

Twins Tell the Tale

Researchers who studied sets of identical twins—siblings who share the exact same genes—were able to show a link between genes and diabetes. But they found that heredity has a stronger link to type 2 diabetes. For example, if one identical twin has type 1 diabetes, then the other twin is a little more likely than most people to develop the disease. But if one twin has type 2 diabetes, then the other twin has a *much* higher chance of developing the disease.

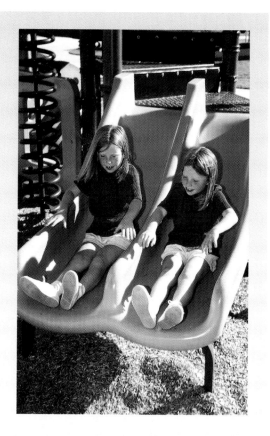

If one twin has type 2 diabetes, the other twin has a good chance of developing the disease.

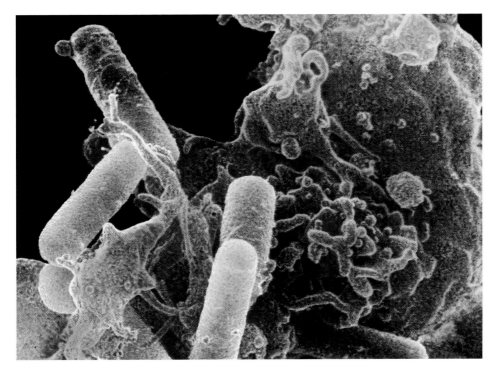

A white blood cell (orange) is attacking bacteria (blue).

Researchers have found that some viruses (tiny disease germs), such as those that cause the common cold or mumps, may damage the pancreas. When you get sick, your body normally does a good job defending itself. Germs are quickly spotted by special defending cells and these cells fight off the germ. But the body's defending cells may make a mistake and attack islet cells, too. Insulin-producing cells are damaged, and the pancreas can no longer produce enough insulin to keep the blood sugar level under control. This can lead to type 1 diabetes.

Activity 1: Diabetes Definitions

Find out how well you understand diabetes.
Choose the **best** definition for each word.

1. Islets

2. Pancreas

3. Glucose

4. Starch

5. Insulin

6. Glucagon

7. Glucose monitor

8. Insulin shock

9. Diabetic coma

A. Hormone that lowers blood sugar level

B. Tests blood sugar level

C. Serious reaction caused by ketones

D. Hormone-producing cells in the pancreas

E. Simple sugar

F. Complex carbohydrate

G. Organ that produces insulin and glucagon

H. Hormone that raises blood sugar level

I. Serious reaction to too much insulin

Testing for Diabetes

The medical name for diabetes is diabetes mellitus. Mellitus, which means honey, is used in the name because sugar that passes out into the urine gives it a sweet taste. Years ago, doctors used to actually taste a patient's urine to make a **diagnosis**. These days, doctors have tests and machines that can do the testing for them.

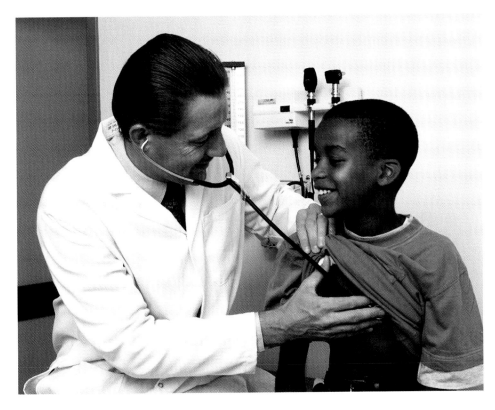

It is very important to see a doctor right away if you think you may have diabetes.

Testing for Glucose

Urine tests were used in the past to detect diabetes, but doctors now depend more on blood tests. Urine tests do a poor job of showing your blood glucose level. Glucose doesn't "spill over" into the urine until there is already quite a lot of glucose in the blood.

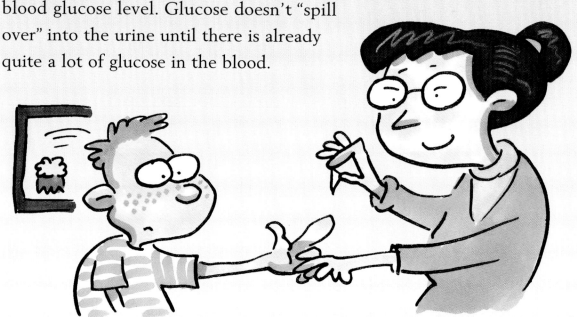

If you have symptoms that suggest diabetes, you should see a doctor right away. The easiest way for the doctor to detect diabetes is to do a **plasma glucose test**. This test measures how much glucose is in the blood. Blood can be taken through a needle in your arm or even with a little finger prick. Only a small amount of blood is needed.

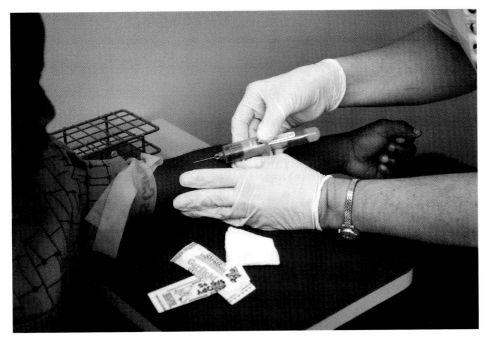

A doctor or nurse will remove some blood from your arm to test for diabetes.

Although a glucose test can be done at any time of the day, the results will vary greatly depending on when you last ate. This is because eating raises the blood sugar level. A **fasting plasma glucose test** is a better way to test for diabetes. This test is taken early in the morning, before you have eaten anything. Normally after fasting, a person's blood contains less than 110 milligrams of glucose in each deciliter of blood. But a person with diabetes will have a fasting glucose level that is more than 126 mg/dl. Two fasting glucose tests taken on different days are needed to make a diagnosis of diabetes.

The **_glucose tolerance test_** gives more information on how the body handles sugar. The blood sugar is first tested after fasting. Then a patient drinks a concentrated sugar solution. Blood samples are then taken several times over the next three hours and tested for the amount of glucose. At first, the glucose drink makes the blood sugar level rise, but then the level falls. It is usually back to normal after two or three hours. In people with diabetes, the blood sugar goes up much higher after taking the glucose drink, and it falls more slowly. Even after three hours it may still be high.

Once diabetes is diagnosed, treatment should begin right away. As you know, high glucose levels can lead to serious problems.

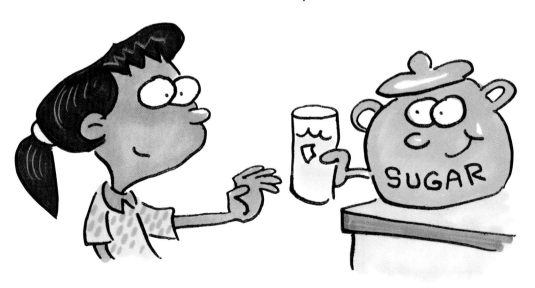

Treating Diabetes

Since diabetes is caused by a lack of working insulin, it makes sense that a common treatment is to put this hormone into the body. Unfortunately, there is no insulin pill or liquid you can drink. Instead, insulin

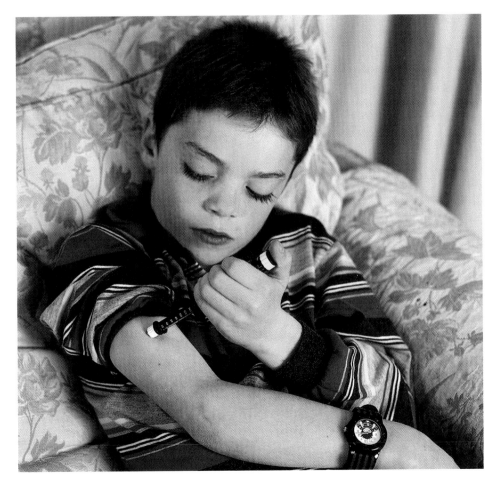

This boy is giving himself an insulin injection.

must be **injected**. The needle doesn't squirt insulin directly into the blood. Instead, it goes into a muscle or fatty area. That way the body can absorb the hormone more slowly rather than all at once. Some common places for injecting insulin are the thighs, buttocks, belly, or upper arms.

People with type 1 diabetes who do not make any insulin need daily insulin shots to keep their condition under control. But most people can't go to the doctor every single day for shots. That's why there are special kits that allow diabetes patients to give insulin shots in their own homes. Parents usually give insulin shots to their young children with

Did You Know...

Insulin has to be injected into the body because if it were swallowed, most of it would be destroyed by digestive juices. Then it would not be able to do its job effectively.

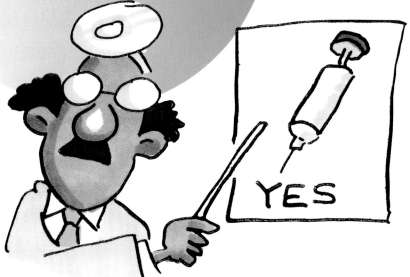

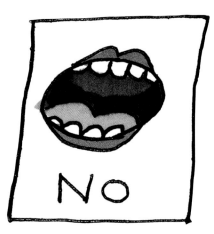

YES NO

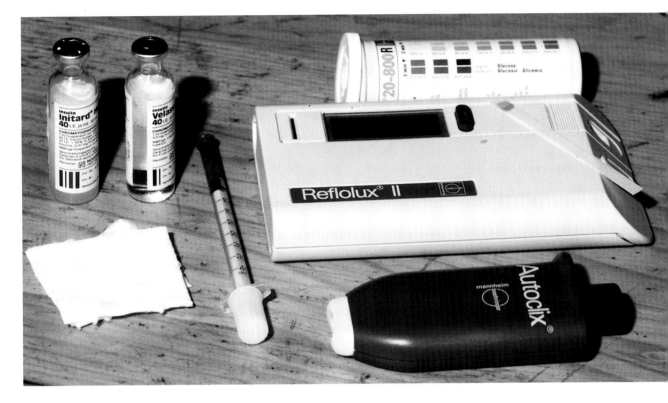

diabetes, but older kids can learn to give insulin shots to themselves. Kids with diabetes say that, at first, it can be a little scary giving yourself a shot. But after awhile, it becomes a routine like getting dressed or brushing your teeth.

There are some devices that make taking insulin easier. An automatic injector can shoot the needle into your skin so that you hardly feel it. It's quick and easy. Insulin pens are a popular choice too. An insulin pen looks just like a regular pen, but instead of a writing tip,

Diabetics use special kits that have all the tools they need to give themselves insulin shots.

An insulin pen
is another way
of injecting
insulin into
the body.

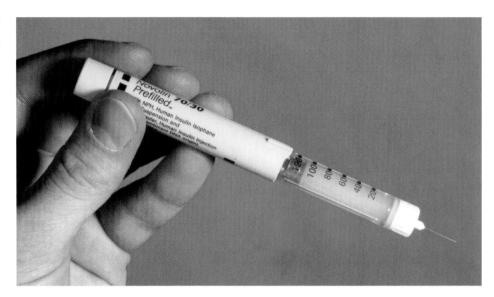

it has a needle. And instead of an ink cartridge, it contains an insulin cartridge. Insulin pens are simple to use and can be carried around in a pocket. Jet injectors give insulin without even using a needle. The insulin is shot out so fast that it goes right into the skin.

Researchers have been working on an insulin inhaler, which delivers the hormone by squirting it into the nose. They expect the device to be available in the near future. This is especially good news for people who don't like needles. Health experts say that people with type 1 diabetes may still need injections, but using an insulin inhaler may reduce the number of injections.

Insulin shots need to be given several times every day, the way insulin is released from a healthy pancreas.

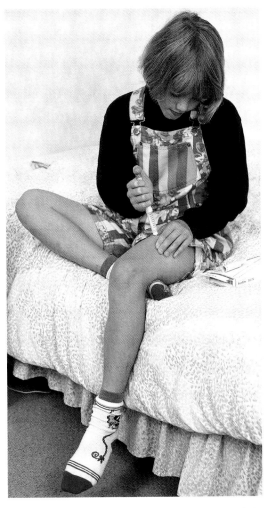

It is usually best to get an insulin shot before a meal.

Normally, a person's body produces insulin in response to food, which boosts the blood glucose levels. As the blood glucose levels fall between meals, so does the insulin production. To keep blood glucose levels normal, people with diabetes should receive insulin three times a day before each meal and another one at night before bed.

Several different kinds of insulin help to control the blood glucose level. Short-acting insulin works quickly and is good for taking before a meal. Long- or medium-acting insulin takes longer to start working but lasts longer. The nighttime injection keeps the glucose level normal during sleep.

Insulin Pump

Having to inject yourself several times a day may seem like a hassle. So how would you like a device that does it for you automatically? An insulin pump is about the size of a beeper and can clip onto your belt or be carried in your pocket. It is attached to a flexible plastic tube and a needle that is inserted under the skin and taped in place. A tiny built-in computer operates a pump that sends exactly the right amount of insulin into your body. You can also deliver an extra dose just before a meal. You have to do some experimenting first to figure out the right amount of insulin flow, but researchers are working on devices that also test the amount of glucose in the blood and adjust the insulin dose automatically—just like a real pancreas.

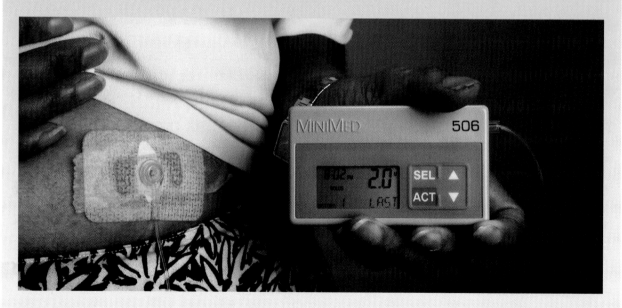

An insulin pump automatically delivers insulin to a patient throughout the day.

Many people who have type 2 diabetes don't need daily insulin injections. They may take pills to keep their blood sugar under control. The pills do not contain insulin. They contain a drug that helps the body make more insulin or use insulin more effectively.

Exercise and diet are also very important in keeping diabetes under control. You burn sugar for energy when you exercise, and the blood glucose level decreases. Exercise also burns up food that might otherwise be stored in the body as fat. It helps you to avoid obesity, which can make diabetes symptoms worse.

What about diet? You might think that someone with diabetes should never eat sugar or any sweet foods, but it is more complicated than that. Everybody needs *some* sugar, but the body can get it from starches and other foods. The problem with eating candy or other high-sugar foods is that much of their sugar doesn't need to be digested. It goes right into the blood, and the blood glucose level shoots up. Then you need more insulin—fast! Starches and other complex carbohydrates, such as those found in bread,

Activity 2: Sugar vs. Starch

Making models of sugars and starches can help you understand how your body uses food for energy. You'll need construction paper, scissors, and tape. Cut out fifteen strips of paper, each measuring 1/2 inch (about 1 cm) wide. Curve one strip into a loop and tape the ends together. This is like a glucose molecule. It is a simple sugar. Now make two more strips into loops, but before you close the second one, link it with the first. This is like a sucrose (table sugar) molecule, which is made of two simple sugars, linked together. Now take all the rest of the strips you cut out, and make them into a chain.

Only simple sugars can be used directly for energy. Sucrose and starches have to be broken down into simple sugars to supply energy. Unpeel the tape on a link of the sucrose molecule and pull it out of the other link. This is like what the body has to do to get energy from sucrose. Now take one link at a time off the "starch" chain. Imagine how long it would take for a real starch molecule! That is why complex carbohydrates provide energy at a much slower rate.

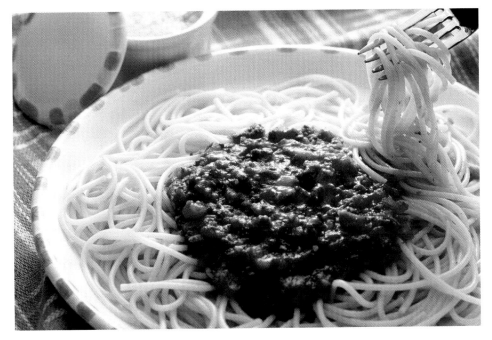

Pasta is a complex carbohydrate that delivers glucose to the body slowly.

pasta, or rice, do need to be digested. So they send glucose into the blood slowly and gradually.

Researchers have been working on other promising diabetes treatments. Some patients with type 1 diabetes have received pancreas transplants. Part or all of a healthy pancreas is placed in a patient. People with successful pancreas transplants may not need to take insulin anymore. The problem with getting a transplant, however, is that the body may identify the new pancreas as foreign and reject it. The body will then attack it, and make the person sick. Doctors have to give patients special drugs to make sure this does not happen.

Living With Diabetes

There is no cure for diabetes at this time. It is a condition that a person has to live with every single day.

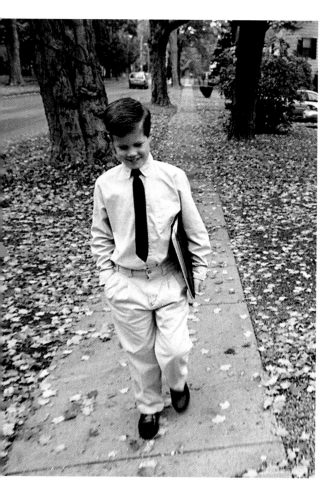

But diabetes can be controlled, and people who have it can live long, healthy lives.

A health care specialist can help patients come up with a good plan that is just right for that individual. What may be good for one person may not be good for another. For example, the amount of insulin needs to be adjusted according to the person's individual needs.

Monitoring glucose is an important part of living with diabetes. People with diabetes need to check

A diabetes patient is collecting donations for the American Diabetes Foundation.

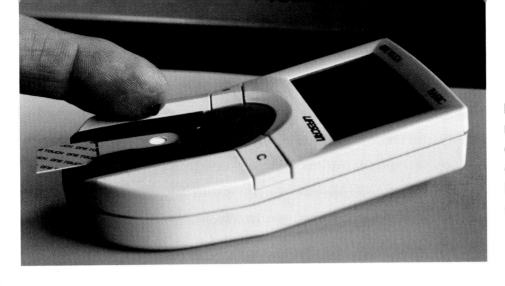

Home glucose monitoring devices make checking blood sugar easy.

their blood glucose levels several times a day to see how well their condition is being controlled. This helps to give a better idea of how much insulin is needed.

Blood glucose monitors are devices that can measure blood sugar levels in a matter of minutes. Regular use of a monitor helps you to figure out how much insulin you need.

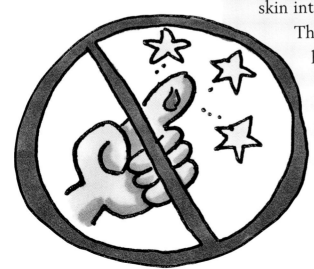

"Ouchless" Monitors

Many people—especially kids—don't like pricking their fingers several times every day. So researchers have been trying to create glucose monitors that don't need to prick the skin at all. The GlucoWatch, worn on the wrist, uses a tiny electric current to draw fluid through the skin into a pad, where glucose is measured. The amount of electricity is too small to hurt or even tingle. Another "ouchless" monitor, now being developed, uses ultrasound (sound too high-pitched for humans to hear) to measure the glucose levels in the body.

Blood sugar is tested by pricking a finger or earlobe and placing a drop of blood into a small portable machine that provides a digital readout of blood sugar levels. Glucose monitoring is very important because it helps you to avoid serious problems that may develop.

Missing doses of insulin, eating too much, or getting an infection or injury may lead to a serious condition called **diabetic coma**. Headaches, tiredness, confusion, stomach pain, and breathing problems may develop as **ketones** build up. Eventually the person may even lose consciousness. Quick emergency care is needed to diagnose and treat the problem.

Sometimes people with diabetes take too much insulin by mistake, causing a low blood sugar level. This can be dangerous. Too much glucose will

Did You Know...

The breath of people with uncontrolled diabetes often has a fruity smell. This is due to ketones, chemicals that are formed when fat is burned for energy. Too many ketones can poison body cells.

High and Low

Here are a couple of handy terms you may hear people use when they talk about diabetes: People whose glucose level is higher than normal have a condition called **hyperglycemia**. **Hypoglycemia** is a lower-than-normal glucose level.

go out of the blood, and not enough will go to the brain. The brain needs a lot of energy and, without enough glucose, it won't work properly. If the blood glucose level falls too low, **insulin shock** may result. The person may feel chilly, sweaty, hungry, nervous, and irritable. The person may even faint. Insulin shock is a dangerous condition that needs immediate emergency care.

Sometimes you can get a bad reaction even if you take the right amount of insulin. This might happen if you skip a meal. When you don't eat at the usual time, your blood sugar level goes down. But if you have diabetes and take insulin, you may already have taken your scheduled insulin shot. The insulin was supposed to bring your blood sugar down to normal after a meal. But if you don't eat, there will be no extra glucose in your blood. Instead, insulin will take away some of the sugar your brain needs.

Exercise burns up glucose, so exercising more than usual can also cause the blood sugar level to fall very low. Eating snacks between meals and before exercising can help you to avoid an insulin reaction.

Many people with diabetes carry around a quick fix to correct low blood sugar. If they feel dizzy and sick and think they might be getting an insulin reaction, they eat hard candy or take a sweet drink, such as orange juice or soda. The extra sugar goes right into the blood and brings the level back to normal. Children with diabetes should talk to their teachers about bringing snacks to class so they can avoid blood sugar level problems.

It's a good idea to wear a medical identification bracelet or necklace and to carry an I.D. card in case of an emergency. Information on your illness and what to do in case of an insulin reaction, as well as your name and the name and number of someone to contact, can save your life.

A medical identification bracelet alerts doctors that you have diabetes in case you are too sick to tell them.

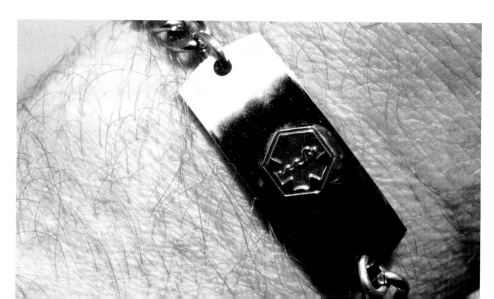

Gl●ssary

carbohydrates—starches and sugars, the body's main energy sources

diabetes—a condition in which insulin is not produced or does not properly control the body's use and storage of sugar, resulting in abnormally high amounts of glucose in the blood; extra glucose may also spill over into the urine

diabetic coma—a serious condition due to a lack of enough insulin. Headache, tiredness, stomach pains, and a loss of consciousness may develop.

diagnosis—identifying a condition from its signs and symptoms

digest—the process by which food is broken down into smaller parts that the body can use

fasting plasma glucose test—a diagnostic test in which the blood glucose level is measured. It has to be taken early in the morning before eating.

genes—chemicals inside each cell that carry inherited traits

gestational diabetes—a type of diabetes that appears in some women during pregnancy, then disappears after the baby is born

glucagon—a hormone that raises the amount of sugar in the blood

glucose—the most common kind of sugar in the blood that the body uses for energy

glucose tolerance test—a test for diabetes in which a person drinks a glucose solution after fasting and the blood sugar is measured several times over the next three hours

hormone—a chemical that helps to control the body's activities

hyperglycemia—a higher-than-normal blood sugar level

hypoglycemia—a lower-than-normal blood sugar level

inherited—passed on by genes from parents to children

injected—sent into the body through a hollow needle

insulin—a hormone that lowers the amount of sugar in the blood and increases the storage of sugar in the liver

insulin resistance—a condition in which the cells are unable to use insulin effectively

insulin shock—a reaction to too much insulin in the blood. Dizziness, confusion, and unconsciousness may develop as the blood sugar level falls.

islets—clusters of insulin-producing cells scattered through the pancreas

ketones—chemicals that are formed when the body burns fat

obesity—condition of being extremely overweight

pancreas—an organ that produces hormones, such as insulin and glucagon, which help to control the amount of glucose in the blood; it also makes digestive juices

plasma glucose test—a diagnostic test in which the blood glucose level is measured; it can be taken at any time of the day

secrete—to release or send out

starch—a food substance found in bread, potatoes, and pasta that the body breaks down into sugars

urinate—to pass liquid body wastes (urine) produced by the kidneys

Learning More

Books

American College of Physicians. *Home Medical Guide to Diabetes*. New York: Dorling Kindersley, Ltd., 2000.

American Diabetes Association. *American Diabetes Association Complete Guide to Diabetes*. New York: Bantam Books, 2000.

American Diabetes Association. *Diabetes A to Z: What You Need to Know About Diabetes—Simply Put*. Alexandria, VA: American Diabetes Association, 1997.

The Dr. Wellbook Collection. *Bear Spot Learns a Lot: Growing up with Diabetes*. Gladstone, NJ: Tim Peters and Company, Inc., 1997.

Gosselin, Kim. *Taking Diabetes to School*. Valley Park, MO: JayJo Books, LLC, 1998.

Silverstein, Alvin, Virginia, & Robert. *Diabetes*. Hillside, NJ: Enslow Publishers, Inc., 1994.

Tonnessen, Diana. *Diabetes: 50 Essential Things to Do*. New York: Penguin Putnam, Inc., 1996.

Organizations and Online Sites

American Diabetes Association
National Service Center
P.O. Box 25757
1660 Duke Street
Alexandria, VA 22314
(800) ADA-DISC (232-3472)
http://www.diabetes.org

Diabetes
http://www.jdf.org/jdfliving/pages/
This site, provided by Juvenile Diabetes Foundation International, includes many links on various aspects of diabetes. One of the links includes a list of diabetes books for kids and adults.

Joslin Diabetes Center
One Joslin Place
Boston, MA 02215
(617) 732-2400

Juvenile Diabetes Foundation International
120 Wall Street, 19th floor
New York, NY 10005
(800) 223-1138
http://www.jdfcure.com

National Institute of Diabetes and Digestive and Kidney Diseases
One Information Way
Bethesda, MD 20892-3560
(301) 654-3327
http://www.niddk.hih.gov/health/diabetes/diabetes.htm

Index

About the Authors

Dr. Alvin Silverstein is a professor of biology at the College of Staten Island of the City University of New York. **Virginia B. Silverstein** is a translator of Russian scientific literature. The Silversteins first worked together on a research project at the University of Pennsylvania. Since then, they have produced 6 children and more than 180 published books for young people.

Laura Silverstein Nunn, a graduate of Kean College, has been helping with her parents' books since her high-school days. She is the coauthor of more than 50 books on diseases and health, science concepts, endangered species, and pets. Laura lives with her husband Matt and their young son Cory in a rural New Jersey town not far from her childhood home.